Postnatal and Neonatal Midwifery Skills

Survival Guide

2nd Edition

Alison Edwards

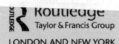

Routledge
Taylor & Francis Group

LONDON AND NEW YORK

Second edition published 2021
by Routledge
2 Park Square, Milton Park, Abingdon, Oxon, OX14 4RN

and by Routledge
52 Vanderbilt Avenue, New York, NY 10017

Routledge is an imprint of the Taylor & Francis Group, an informa business

First edition published by Pearson Education Limited 2012

British Library Cataloguing-in-Publication Data
A catalogue record for this book is available from the British Library

Library of Congress Cataloging-in-Publication Data
A catalog record has been requested for this book

ISBN: 978-1-138-38891-8 (pbk)
ISBN: 978-0-429-42428-1 (ebk)

Typeset in Helvetica
by Cenveo® Publisher Services
Printed in Canada

contents

Figures

Tables

Abbreviations

TIP

Many abbreviations are used in midwifery; however, officially only those accepted by your individual Trust should be used!

APH	antepartum haemorrhage
BD	twice daily
BMI	body mass index
BP	blood pressure
BPM	beats per minute
C/O	care of/complaining of
CAF	Common Assessment Framework
CRL	crown rump length
CTG	cardiotocograph
DOB	date of birth
DV	domestic violence
DVT	deep vein thrombosis
EBL	estimated blood loss
EDD	estimated due date/estimated date of delivery
FBC	fluid balance chart or full blood count
FBS	fetal blood sample
FD	forceps delivery
FH	fundal height

FHHR	fetal heart heard and regular/reactive
FL	femur length
FM	fetal movements
FSE	fetal scalp electrode
G	gravida (the number of pregnancies)
G & S	group and save
H/O	history of
Hb	haemoglobin
HC	head circumference
HELLP	haemolysis, elevated liver enzymes and low platelets
HVS	high vaginal swab
IUCD	intrauterine contraceptive device
IUD	intrauterine death
IUGR	intrauterine growth restriction
IVI	intravenous infusion
LBW	low birth weight
LFT	liver function tests
LMWH	Low molecular weight heparin
LOA	left occipito anterior
LOP	left occipito posterior
LSCS	lower segment caesarean section
MC & S	microscopy and sensitivity
MEW/MEOW	modified early (obstetric) warning score
ML	millilitre

MLC	Midwifery-led care
MSU	Mid-stream urine
NBM	nil by mouth
NG	nasogastric
NNU	neonatal unit
NVB	normal vaginal birth
OA	occipito anterior
OP	occipito posterior
P	parity (the number of births over 24 weeks)
PO	per oral
PR	per rectum
PV	per vagina
RDS	respiratory distress syndrome
ROA	right occipito anterior
ROP	right occipito posterior
SB	stillbirth
SCBU	special care baby unit
SGA	small for gestational age
SIDS	sudden infant death syndrome
SROM	spontaneous rupture of membranes
TDS	three times daily
TPR	temperature, pulse and respirations
TTN	transient tachypnea of the newborn

U & E	urea and electrolytes
USS	ultrasound scan
UTI	urinary tract infection
VBAC	vaginal birth after caesarean
VE	vaginal examination
Xmatch	cross-match

Anatomy and physiology

■ FETAL CIRCULATION

Figure 1 The fetal circulation

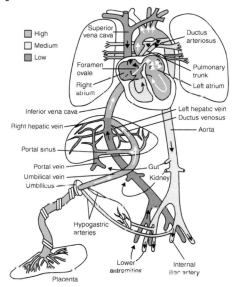

Source: Reproduced with permission from. Fernandes CJ. Physiologic transition from intrauterine to extrauterine life. In: UpToDate, Basow, DS (Ed), UpToDate, Waltham, MA 2012. Copyright © 2012 UpToDate, Inc. For more information visit www.uptodate.com.

Four main structures which differ from adult circulation

- **Ductus venosus** – directs oxygenated blood from the umbilical vein to the inferior vena cava.
- **Foramen ovale** – an opening between the atria of the heart which allows blood to bypass the pulmonary circulation.
- **Ductus arteriosus** – diverts blood away from the pulmonary artery back into the aorta.
- **Two hypogastric arteries** – direct blood from the lower extremities back through the umbilical arteries to the placenta.

Extra features

- Red blood cells are greater in number and larger than adult blood cells.
- The life span of these red blood cells is shorter.
- Fetal haemoglobin has greater oxygen-carrying capacity.

At birth

- Changes in temperature and compression of the chest wall during the birth stimulate the baby to take a breath.
- Blood is drawn towards the alveoli in the lungs and then returned to the left atrium of the heart. This lowers the pressure in the right atrium and raises the pressure in the left atrium, causing the foramen ovale to be covered by a flap of tissue. Blood is now directed into the right ventricle and out to the lungs.
- Blood bypasses the ductus arteriosus and the direction of blood circulating reverses. The ductus arteriosus eventually closes to form a ligament.

- The separation of the umbilical cord cuts off the placental blood supply further, lowering the pressure in the right atrium. Blood can no longer circulate through the hypogastric arteries, umbilical vessels and ductus venosus. These structures eventually form ligaments.

■ INVOLUTION

- The process whereby the uterus returns to its pre-pregnancy size of 60 grams. By 10 days post birth the uterus is usually no longer palpable above the pelvic brim.
- **Autolysis** – proteolytic enzymes digest the muscle cells that are no longer required. Phagocytes remove the debris.
- **Ischaemia** – blood supply is reduced to the decidua due to constriction of the spiral arteries after birth. The decidua therefore dies and is shed as lochia. By 6 weeks post birth the endometrium has reformed.
- **Contraction and retraction** – oxytocin continues to be released (especially if the mother is breastfeeding); therefore contraction and retraction of the myometrium continues.

■ LOCHIA

- The vaginal loss following the birth.
- 3–4 days post birth = RUBRA (red from blood from placental site, decidual tissue, vernix and amniotic fluid).
- 5–9 days post birth = SEROSA (pink then brown from reduced blood loss, serum and leucocytes).
- 10–28 days post birth = ALBA (yellow/white from cervical mucus, debris and leucocytes).

■ BREAST

Figure 2 The anatomy of the breast

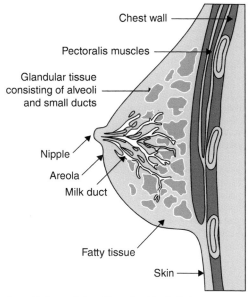

Source: http://www.celtnet.org.uk/cancer/breast-function.html.

Bereavement – dealing with the loss of a baby

Unfortunately, babies continue to be stillborn, die in utero or die within days of the birth. It proves to be an extremely difficult time for the families but also for the staff involved. There are, however, a number of activities that need to be undertaken. Some of these may help with the emotional distress.

- Encourage though don't force the parents to hold their baby and spend some time with them – this amount of time should be dictated by the parents themselves.
- Sitting and listening/discussing events.
- Respond to the signals – every set of parents will deal differently with grief. Act professionally but sensitively and use understandable terminology.
- Take foot and hand prints, locks of hair, photographs, and provide additional identity bracelets. Parents may not wish to take these away with them immediately, so store them in the notes as they may ask for them at a later date.
- Siblings need support too. Textbooks are available which provide strategies for this
- Handle the baby gently – help the parents wash and dress their baby if they wish or do it for them.
- Discussing the funeral arrangements, while difficult, can help provide a focus. Hospitals usually have their own policies on this and will often also hold memorial services.
- Invite faith leaders/chaplains to visit if appropriate.
- Parents often ask the question *why* it happened. It isn't always possible to answer this question, but a post-mortem and a series of screening tests are

offered/carried out with consent which may answer the question. An appointment to return to discuss the results with an obstetrician is required.

- All stillbirths and neonatal deaths must be reported – relevant forms will be found on each delivery suite.
- A death certificate should be completed and passed to the parents. The parents will need to register the birth and death with the Registrar of Births and Deaths within 42 days of the baby's delivery. In Scotland the time limit is 21 days and in Northern Ireland the time limit is 5 days. If the parents are married the registrar will need details of both parents. If the parents are not married only the details of the mother are required, but the father can give his details.
- Postnatal care should continue as normal for the woman.
- Women can be offered medication to suppress lactation.
- The baby can be placed in the hospital mortuary until tests are completed and the baby is collected for funeral or cremation. Until then, parents should be able to visit the baby in the chapel of rest as they wish. Alternatively, some units have refrigerated cots which enable the baby to remain with its parents.
- You will need to inform the woman's GP and cancel any referrals to the health visitors.
- Make sure that all documentation is complete.

Blood values

Electrolytes

- Sodium (Na)   134–146mmol/L
- Potassium (K)   3.4–5.0mmol/L
- Glucose   3.0–7.8mmol/L
                                             3.9–6.2mmol/L (fasting)
- Urea (age-dependent)   4.0–8.0mmol/L
- Creatinine (age-dependent)   0.05–0.12mmol/L
- Total protein   63–78g/L
- Albumin   35–45g/L
- Globulin   25–45g/L
- Bilirubin total   3–17pmol/L
- Alkaline phosphatase (ALP)   35–150U/L
- Gamma GT   5–40U/L
- Alanine transaminase (ALT)   1–45U/L
- Aspartate transaminase (AST)   1–36U/L
- Calcium (Ca)   2.15–2.60mmol/L
- Total cholesterol   <200mg/dL
                                             <5.5mmol/L (fasting)

Blood gases

- pH   7.36–7.44
- pCO_2 36–44mmHg
- PaO_2 85–100mmHg
- Bicarbonate   22–29mmol/L
- Base excess   −2 to +2mmol/L
- Oxygen saturation   94–98%

Thyroid function tests

Thyroid-stimulating hormone (TSH) 1–11mU/L.

Haematology

- WBC $4.5–11 \times 10^9$/L
- RBC   Female $4.2–5.4 \times 10^9$/L
- Hb   Female 120–160g/L
- Mean cell volume (MCV)   80–100fL
- Platelets $150–400 \times 10^9$/L
- Lymphocytes   25–33%

Bottle feeding

■ STERILISATION OF FEEDING EQUIPMENT

Cold water sterilising

- Either a bought sterilising unit or a clean bucket/plastic container with a lid can be used. The bucket or container should be deep enough to submerge the equipment entirely.
- Dissolve a sterilising tablet in cold water to the suggested ratio on the packet.
- Bottles should be rinsed clear of old milk before re-sterilisation – use a bottle brush if needed.
- Submerge the bottles and teats, etc., ensuring there are no air bubbles inside.
- Use the equipment provided with the bought unit or something, such as a heavy plate, to keep the bottles and other equipment completely under the solution.
- It takes around 30 minutes to sterilise.
- Take out bottles and teats only when required. Shake out any excess solution, or rinse off the fluid with cool, boiled water (though this isn't compulsory).
- Change the solution every 24 hours.

Boiling

- Bottles should be suitable for this.
- Place in a large pan with a lid or cover. Use the pan exclusively for this purpose.
- Fill the pan with water and submerge all the feeding equipment completely. Make sure there are no trapped air

bubbles inside the bottles and teats, then cover the pan and boil for at least 10 minutes.

- Keep the pan's cover on until you need to use the equipment.

Electric steam sterilising

- Takes between 8 to 12 minutes, plus cooling time.
- Can keep bottles sterilised for up to 6 hours if left in the steriliser with the lid closed.
- Bottles, teats and other equipment should be placed with their openings downwards.
- Check all equipment is safe to use in a steam steriliser before using.

Microwaves

- Check that bottles can be sterilised in the microwave.
- Takes around 90 seconds to sterilise a single bottle.
- Do not seal the bottles during microwaving.
- Special steamers are available for microwave use. These steamers take about 3 to 8 minutes to work plus cooling time, depending on the model and microwave wattage.
- The items also remain sterile for 3 hours if the steriliser lid is kept closed.

Dishwasher sterilising

- Check that equipment is dishwasher safe.
- Use a hot programme of 80°C or more.
- Make up feed immediately because bacteria can begin to form as soon as the bottle is removed from the dishwasher.

■ MAKING UP FORMULA FEEDS

- All equipment must have been sterilised, including bottles, teats and teat covers. Leave to drip dry.
- Boil kettle and leave to cool to around 70°C (approximately 15 minutes for 500ml of water).
- Wash hands thoroughly, especially after changing nappies.
- *Always* put the correct amount of water into the bottle first.
- Using the scoop provided with the formula, add the appropriate number of scoops of milk powder. The scoops should be levelled off using a knife. The scoop must not be over- or under filled.
- Place top on bottle and shake the bottle to mix the milk thoroughly.
- Allow to cool further (it should feel lukewarm to the inside of the forearm). If needed, run the bottle under the cold tap.
- It is recommended that feeds should no longer be made up in advance and that any feed should be used within 2 hours. Any leftover feed should be disposed of after 2 hours.

Other tips

- Women on income support who choose to formula feed may be entitled to vouchers to buy milk powder.
- Whey-dominant powders are recommended over casein dominant; however, both can be used from birth.
- Babies who bottle feed are more likely to need winding post feed.
- Weaning should take place after around 6 months.

Breastfeeding

■ PHYSIOLOGY OF LACTATION

Breast changes in pregnancy

- From the sixth week of pregnancy oestrogen influences the growth of the ducts and tubules in the breast. Progesterone, prolactin and human placental lactogen (HPL) cause enlargement of the alveoli.
- By 12 weeks the Montgomery's tubercles (sebaceous glands on the areola) secrete lubricants onto the breast surface.
- Colostrum is produced under the influence of HPL and prolactin from 16 weeks' gestation.
- In pregnancy milk production is inhibited by high levels of oestrogen and progesterone. These levels drop dramatically once the placenta is delivered, enabling prolactin levels to increase and milk production to commence.

Milk production

- Prolactin-releasing hormone (from the hypothalamus) stimulates prolactin (from the anterior pituitary) production which in turn stimulates the acini cells of the breasts to produce milk. Prolactin release peaks towards the end of feeds.
- When suckling stops, prolactin-inhibiting factor (produced by the hypothalamus and secreted in the breast milk) is released to block milk production when the feed is complete.
- Subsequently milk production works on a supply-and-demand principle.

- The cycle is initiated by stimulus (e.g. by the baby suckling). This stimulus results in oxytocin being released by the posterior pituitary. Oxytocin contracts the cells in the alveoli forcing milk down the milk ducts and into the baby's mouth, aided by the baby's sucking motion. (A neurohormonal reflex or the 'Let down reflex'.)

Tips

- Encouraging an initial breastfeed and skin-to-skin within the first hour of birth will greatly improve the success of subsequent breastfeeding.
- Prolactin levels increase at night to prepare the body for feeds the following day, so it is normal for babies to feed through the night.
- Women opting to formula feed will produce milk initially but need to avoid stimulating the breasts to aid cessation of milk production.
- Women with HIV may be discouraged from breastfeeding due to possible transmission.

■ ADVANTAGES OF BREASTFEEDING

For the baby

- Protects from leukaemia, rotavirus and gastrointestinal infections.
- Protects against respiratory problems, including asthma, and against urinary problems.
- Reduces chance of developing eczema and food allergies.
- Aids mouth and jaw development and teeth alignment.
- Reduces the likelihood of obesity in childhood.
- Reduces the risk of ear infections.

- Helps prevent necrotising enterocolitis, especially in premature infants.
- Thought to reduce the risk of SIDS.
- Maternal antibodies are passed on to baby to aid immunity.

For the woman

- Protects against breast and ovarian cancers.
- May help with postmenopausal bone density.
- Exclusively breastfeeding can provide effective contraception.
- Aids weight loss.
- Helps bonding and overall feeling of well-being.
- Breast milk is produced on demand and at the correct temperature.
- Breastfeeding is convenient and free.

■ STEPS TO AID SUCCESSFUL BREASTFEEDING

1. Units should have a written breastfeeding policy that is routinely communicated to all healthcare staff.
2. Train all healthcare staff in the skills necessary to implement the breastfeeding policy.
3. Inform all pregnant women about the benefits and management of breastfeeding throughout pregnancy.
4. Help mothers initiate breastfeeding soon after birth – use skin-to-skin within the first hour of birth.
5. Show mothers how to breastfeed and how to maintain lactation, even if they are separated from their babies. Take a hands-off approach to help the woman build confidence.

6. Give newborn infants no food or drink other than breast milk, unless medically indicated.

7. Encourage mothers and infants to remain together 24 hours per day. If not possible due to the baby being in a NNU, for example, encourage hand expression and provide the mother with a reminder of her baby.

8. Encourage reciprocal/responsive feeding, as this helps build relationships. Respond to feeding cues, including sucking fingers, opening or smacking mouth, restlessness, crying. Hold the baby close and maintain eye contact. Pace and time feeds to meet the needs of both the mother and baby. The baby will detach when satisfied.

9. Give no artificial teats or dummies to breastfeeding infants.

10. Foster the establishment of breastfeeding support groups and refer women to them on discharge from the hospital or clinic.

Table 1 Signs that the baby is attached correctly and feeding well

- **The baby is held close – tummy to mummy and in line with the nipple. Support shoulders**
- **Large mouthful of breast with bottom lip curled back**
- **More areola seen above than below**
- **Full, rounded cheeks**
- **Rhythmical sucking with small pauses**
- **Chin touches the breast and head free to tilt back**

Source: WHO/UNICEF (2016) *Protecting, Promoting and Supporting Breastfeeding: The Special Role of Maternity Services.* A joint WHO/UNICEF Statement. Geneva: WHO.

■ HAND EXPRESSION

Where women are unable to directly breastfeed their babies (e.g. if the baby is on the neonatal unit), hand expression is recommended. If possible, this should take place 6–8 times during a 24-hour period, including the night. This skill can take some practice but can prove more effective than using breast pumps and is said to produce milk with a higher fat content.

Figure 3 Hand expression

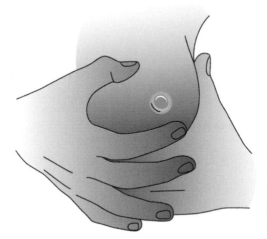

Procedure

- Wash hands (and breasts if needed – some nipple creams need to be wiped away).
- A sterilised container wide enough to sit under the breast to collect the milk is required.
- The woman should be sitting comfortably, well supported and as upright as possible.
- To aid the release of oxytocin, either have the baby nearby or ask the woman to gently massage each breast for about 5 minutes each. Using warm flannels may also help.
- Ask the woman to place her little finger underneath her breast, against her ribs, and use the remaining fingers to support the breast. The thumb needs to be on top, about 2cm or 4cm back from the base of the nipple, depending on breast size and shape. The woman should be feeling for a change in the texture of the breast.
- The hand should be pushed inwards towards the chest wall and the fingers should gently compress the breast tissue in a press-and-release motion towards the nipple.
- This rhythmic motion should be repeated until drops of colostrum or breast milk appear at the nipple. NB: It may take a minute or two for milk to appear. Initially there will be drips followed by squirts of milk as more milk is produced.
- DO NOT drag the fingers and thumb over the skin of the breast, as this may cause damage to the skin.
- Systematically reposition the hand slightly and repeat the movement on different sections of the breast before changing to the other breast.

Breast milk storage

- Milk should be refrigerated as soon as possible but can be kept up to 6 hours at room temperature in a sealed sterile container.
- Milk can be kept towards the back of a fridge for up to 8 days at −4°C, 4 days above −4°C.
- Milk can be kept in a freezer for 3–6 months and in a deep freezer for up to a year.
- Any defrosted milk should not be refrozen. Milk *must* be completely defrosted before use, ideally in the fridge or container run under cool then warm water.

Calculating feed requirements

Babies' feed requirements change on a daily basis. In some cases (e.g. when a baby is admitted to the neonatal unit), it is necessary to calculate the correct amount for the age of the neonate. To do this the following formula is used:

$$\frac{\text{Daily requirement} \times \text{weight in kilograms}}{\text{Number of feeds in 24 hrs}}$$

Examples could be:

Day 0–1 = 60ml per day × 2kg ÷ 8 (this will equate to 3 hourly feeds) = 10ml per feed.

Day 2 = 90ml per day × 2kg ÷ 6 (this equates to 4 hourly feeds) = 30ml per feed.

Day 3 = 120ml per day × 2kg ÷ 6 = 40ml per feed.

Changing stools and number of wet/dirty nappies

- In the first 48 hours 1–2 wet nappies and 1 or more stools.
- From birth to 2 days: stool (meconium) is dark green/black, thick and sticky.
- 3–4 days old: 'changing stools' become a less dark green/brown colour and may have 'seeds' of yellow in it. 3 or more wet nappies and 2 or more stools.
- 5–6 days old: stool is usually yellow. 5 or more wet nappies and 2 or more stools.
- Breastfed babies will continue to pass soft yellow, low-odour stools relatively frequently until about 3–4 weeks. This reduces to a bowel movement every 2–3 days after that.
- Formula-fed babies are more likely to pass paler, more formed stools with a slight odour. These babies are prone to constipation.

Contraception

While having another baby may be the last thing on parents' minds just after giving birth, it is an important role of the midwife to discuss contraception prior to discharge.

It is entirely up to the individual couples when they resume intercourse, and this can be influenced by a number of factors.

The type of contraceptive used is largely personal choice; however, factors including overall health, age and lifestyle can impact upon the options available.

Table 2 Contraception options available

Condom (male)	Free from family planning centres Protects against pregnancy and Sexually Transmitted Diseases (STDs) Most have a spermicidal agent applied NB: the majority are made of latex Can be damaged during application by nails, rings, etc., raising the risk of semen leake
Natural methods	Can involve monitoring temperature/mucus discharge and avoidance of intercourse during fertile times Can be difficult to determine 'safe times'
Diaphragm/cap	Must be measured and fitted Women must wait and use alternative methods until 6–8 weeks postnatal before assessment to ensure an accurate fit

(Continued)

Table 2 (*Continued*)

	Should be inserted prior to intercourse and removed after 6 hours post intercourse Must be used with a spermicide to be effective
Condom (female)	Needs to be inserted before penetration and held in place during penetration If used effectively can be 94% successful in preventing pregnancy and protects against STDs
Intrauterine contraceptive devices (IUCDs)	Come in a variety of shapes and sizes Some contain progesterone The copper content is toxic to sperm and ova Can be uncomfortable to insert, especially in nulliparas women Post birth the woman must wait between 6–8 weeks before fitting Can cause an increase in bleeding initially and discomfort Progesterone-based IUCDs also protect from uterine infection unlike other versions; however, thrush is more common Can remain *in situ* for a number of years Strings may cause discomfort to the male during intercourse High success rate and easily removed

Table 2 (*Continued*)

Combined pill	Tablets or patches containing oestrogen and progesterone which prevents ovulation and alters the cervical mucus
	Must be prescribed – taken for 21 days from start of period followed by a 7-day break for the withdrawal bleed
	Side effects include weight gain, headaches, mood changes and an increased risk of DVT/stroke in obese women
	Not recommended if breastfeeding
	Can be started after 21 days post birth
	Can be less effective if on antibiotics or have diarrhoea and vomiting, but otherwise if taken correctly is 99% effective
Progesterone-only pill	Suitable for breastfeeding women
	Started after 21 days post birth
	Initially may affect the amount and frequency of periods
	Alters the cervical mucus inhibiting sperm transmission
	Must be taken every day at around the same time; therefore not suitable for women who may forget to take it
	Some versions have a wider margin for missed tablets

(*Continued*)

Table 2 (*Continued*)

Injected (e.g. Depo-Provera)	Administered every 3 months and can lead to amenorrhoea Administered after 6 weeks post-partum if not awaiting sterilisation or have had unprotected intercourse Does not affect lactation Can lead to weight gain and depression
Implants	A rod containing slow-release progesterone inserted under the skin in the upper arm under local anaesthetic Can be inserted after 21 days post birth Lasts around 3 years and has a high success rate May lead to amenorrhoea Inhibits ovulation and thickens the cervical mucus
Sterilisation	Tubal ligation (female) or vasectomy (male) Individuals require counselling, as this method is permanent Attempts to reverse these procedures are often unsuccessful Usually undertaken at least 6–8 weeks following birth Small failure rate
Exclusive breastfeeding	The baby must be totally breastfed Effective in the first 6 months post birth The woman should be amenorrhoeic

Cord care

- The umbilical stump will harden and dry through a process of dry gangrene. This is helped by exposure to air.
- As the cord separates (within about 10 days), there may be some sticky residue at the base, which is normal.
- Current evidence recommends leaving the cord outside of the nappy (fold the top of the nappy down) and to leave alone.
- At most, use clean water and cotton wool to remove any contamination.
- Do not apply any powders or creams.
- The cord clamp may or may not be removed once the cord has dried – this depends on Trust policy.

Developmental care

- Complements the high-tech medical and nursing care that occurs on neonatal units.
- Provides care around the needs of the individual.
- Based on the principle of re-creating features of the intrauterine environment, including controlled light and sound, diurnal rhythms, constant temperature, nutrition, tactile and vestibular input (uterine boundaries support posture, tone and movement, calming behaviour).
- Light and noise exposure is kept to a minimum.
- Regular contact with parents is important – massage, touching, holding, kangaroo care encouraged.
- Adequate pain relief is important.
- Careful positioning in a secure environment.
- Environmental temperature is regulated.

Discharge – points for discussion

It is recommended that certain topics are discussed with women prior to their leaving the hospital following their birth. Different Trust policies may vary but these topics could include the following:

- Baby car safety.
- Registering the birth – usually required within 42 days of the birth.
- Contraception.
- Emergency contact numbers.
- Infant feeding.
- Follow-up visits, including a six-week appointment (usually with the GP).
- Signs of deviations from normal.
- Prevention of SIDS.

Drugs for neonates

■ VITAMIN K (PHYTOMENADIONE)

- Given either through midwives' exemption (NMC 2017) or prescribed by a paediatrician. Premature babies or babies below 2.5kg must have a prescription due to a greater risk of kernicterus (Joint Formulary Committee 2020).
- At birth, babies are deficient in vitamin K and are at risk of haemorrhage, including intracranial bleeding, hence administration.
- Consent must be obtained from the parents.
- IM dose – single dose 1mg (0.1ml) after birth

or

- Oral × 1 dose of 2mg (0.2ml) at birth and at 7 days. A third dose is recommended for breastfed babies at 28 days.
- With oral administration there is a risk that babies will spit out some of the medicine, or some may not be absorbed, potentially making it less effective.
- The IM route can cause pain and swelling at the administration site.
- Little evidence is available to support a link between childhood leukaemia and the IM administration of vitamin K.

■ NALOXONE

- No longer in regular use.
- Reversal of neonatal respiratory depression arising from opioid administration to a woman in labour.
- IM injection of 200 micrograms or 10 micrograms/kg. Second doses may be needed due to a short half-life.

- Contraindicated in women who use opioids for recreational purposes.
- Can be given via midwives' exemptions or prescribed.

■ HEPATITIS B IMMUNOGLOBULIN

- Administered IM. 200 units as soon after birth as possible to babies of mothers with Hepatitis B during pregnancy or who are positive for Hepatitis B surface antigen.
- Is considered within the midwives' exemptions (NMC 2017); however, review Trust policy.

■ BCG

- Administered to babies at risk of exposure (e.g. with parents from a high-risk country).
- Intradermal injection of 0.1ml.
- Training is required to administer and must be prescribed by a medical practitioner.

Emergencies

Figure 4 Management of a secondary post-partum haemorrhage

Assess blood loss: is it heavy, offensive, are there large clots?
Palpate the uterus: is it contracted; is it involuting?
Is it tender to palpate?
Assess maternal well-being: is the woman complaining of pain, flu-like symptoms? Is she pale or showing signs of shock?

If yes to to any of the above:
Review delivery records: were the placenta and membranes complete?
Take maternal observations: BP, pulse, temperature and respirations; record on a MEOWS if appropriate.
If lochia is offensive perform an HVS and send for culture and sensitivity.
Refer to a medical practitioner.

Options for management will then depend on severity of symptoms.
These include:
Ultrasound scan for retained products
Bloods for FBC, G & S, and CRP, U& Es and blood cultures
Antibiotics
Fluid replacement: IVI
Admission
Surgery for removal of retained products

■ SECONDARY POST-PARTUM HAEMORRHAGE (PPH)

- Occurs after 24 hours of birth and up to 6 weeks post-partum.
- Relatively uncommon.
- Concluding how much blood loss is considered to be a 2°PPH is subjective. Management will depend on maternal well-being, and whether blood loss is greater than average, with or without clots.
- Most common causes are retained products of conception (RPOC), sub-involution of the uterus or uterine infection.

■ SEPSIS

For more details refer to Knight et al. (2014 to 2019).

- Sepsis remains one of the leading causes of maternal deaths in the UK. Prompt recognition and action in response to signs and symptoms is recommended.
- β Haemolytic Streptococcus A infection and influenza have been identified as a leading cause of sepsis resulting in maternal deaths.

Source: Knight et al. (2019) *Saving Lives, Improving Mother's Care.* Oxford: MBRRACE.

Signs requiring urgent referral by ambulance/immediate review by a doctor

- Pyrexia >38°C – however, hypothermia may also be a sign; remember: a high temperature could be masked by paracetamol/analgesia.

- Continued tachycardia >100bpm.
- Increased respiration rate/breathlessness.
- Abdominal or chest pain.
- Diarrhoea and vomiting – can be misdiagnosed as other conditions (e.g. gastroenteritis).
- Uterine pain/tenderness.
- The woman is feeling unwell, over-anxious; she may have symptoms of flu.
- Leucopenia $<4 \times 10^9$ white blood cells is significant.
- Persistent bleeding and offensive lochia.

NB: Anti-pyrexial medication can mask a high temperature and therefore does not exclude sepsis.

Recommendations

- Educate women regarding the signs and symptoms.
- Women should wash hands before and after using the toilet, changing pads or touching any perineal wounds. This is increasingly important if the woman has been in contact with anyone with a sore throat or has one herself.
- Staff should be trained in the recognition of symptoms and the need for early management.

■ MANAGEMENT (INCLUDING THE SEPSIS 6 BUNDLE)

- Refer to hospital/medical practitioner ASAP. Keeping to treatment in the golden hour is ideal.
- If infection is suspected – USS for retained products +/–evacuation of retained products.
- FBC, CRP and blood cultures if temperature >38°C.
- Serum lactate.
- Throat swabs, high vaginal swab, wound swabs.

- Any other relevant samples (e.g. MSU, sputum, breast milk, perineum, stool).
- High-flow facial oxygen 15 litres.
- Commence intravenous high-dose, broad-spectrum antibiotics without waiting for microbiology results. Change to appropriate antibiotics once pathogen identified. Continue for 7–10 days.
- The baby may also require surface swabs.
- Regularly record vital signs – commence MEOWS and fluid balance chart.
- Ensure the baby is cared for or transferred with the mother.
- HDU/ITU care if needed.
- Help with the baby and feeding.

■ SEPTIC SHOCK

Arterial hypertension that is refractory to fluid resuscitation. Fluid overload can lead to fatal pulmonary or cerebral oedema and should therefore be avoided.

Senior anaesthetic input is vital alongside liaison with a critical care team.

Clear accurate records of fluid balance are vital!

Fluid balance

Fluid balance is maintaining the correct amount of fluid in the body through the amount of fluid intake and that which is excreted.

Around 52% of the body weight is from fluid in a non-pregnant woman. During pregnancy an increase in circulating volume of up to 50% alongside retention of fluid, leading to oedema, can affect fluid balance. There are a number of factors that will cause fluid loss and gain in childbearing women.

Loss

- Vomiting (e.g. during labour or from hyperemesis in pregnancy).
- Blood loss from the birth, perineal trauma or operative procedures.
- Sweating/fever.
- Haemorrhage (e.g. post-partum haemorrhage).
- Diarrhoea.

Gain

- Oedema/fluid retention.
- Pre-eclampsia/eclampsia.
- Renal failure.
- High sodium intake.
- Over-infusion of intravenous fluids.

■ RECORDING FLUID BALANCE

Recording fluid balance is usually required for women who are on a high dependency unit (e.g. due to pre-eclampsia or those who have undergone a caesarean section/surgery).

It is usually undertaken alongside vital observations, including blood pressure, pulse, respiration and temperature. High-risk women may also have a central venous pressure (CVP) line sited for more accurate measurements of circulatory function. (CVP is a measurement of pressure in the right atrium of the heart.) These measurements can alter in response to fluid loss or gain (e.g. too little circulating fluid will lead to a weak, thready pulse).

Alongside the above – accurate recordings on a fluid balance chart of all fluids in and out are required. Output of urine is relatively easy to measure, especially if a catheter is *in situ*. Urine may be measured 1 hourly or every time the catheter bag is emptied. Alternatively, women can use a bedpan or bowl to collect any urine passed. Measuring input is less straightforward. Drinking vessels can vary considerably in size; therefore finding out the correct volume is important. Cans and bottled fluids usually have the volume on the packaging. Most intravenous fluids are administered via pumps or have a specified amount prescribed.

Blood tests such as urea and electrolytes, glucose, magnesium and calcium can also indicate whether there are any fluid balance problems.

The totals for input and output should be calculated after a 12- or 24-hour period. The two resulting figures should be relatively the same. Marked discrepancies must be acted upon.

Pre-eclamptic women are at particular risk of fluid retention. It may be necessary to restrict their fluid intake to 85ml/hr. This includes any infused fluids, oral fluids and any medication administered in liquid form.

Hypoglycaemia in the newborn

- More likely in babies who have IUGR or diabetic mothers, are pre-term or have suffered fetal distress.
- A blood sugar of <2.6mmol/L is considered low.
- Signs include poor tone, mottled, pale skin, lethargy, poor feeding, jittering – if severe or prolonged can lead to cyanosis, hypoxia or death.

Management

- Feed immediately, and at regular intervals after that (e.g. 2–3 times hourly).
- Blood sugar samples should be taken 1 hour after each feed.
- Refer to a paediatrician.
- Document.

Modified Obstetric Early Warning System (MEOWS)

- Designed for use on all women but especially those who are high risk.
- Designed to alert staff to act upon any deviations from the normal.
- Regular observations, including vital signs, are plotted and any results falling outside accepted ranges (in some cases within the amber or red sections or in some cases a score) should trigger a referral to medical staff.

Neonatal examination

Alongside the initial examination after birth and the check undertaken by the paediatric team (or appropriately trained midwife) babies are regularly examined during the postnatal period. This usually takes place during the same visits as the postnatal check for the mother. The following list covers aspects of both the initial and subsequent examinations.

Procedure

- Make sure the examination takes place in a warm, draught-free environment and in good light.
- Gain consent from the mother and wash hands.
- If in hospital – check there are two identity labels and security bracelet *in situ*.
- Assess overall well-being – tone, response to handling, alertness.
- Discuss feeding patterns with the mother.
- Assess skin colour for any jaundice, paleness, cyanosis, port wine stains, birthmarks, signs of trauma, café au lait spots, skin tags, milia and signs of infection (rashes, white spots). Remember: the skin of a newborn is thin and functionally immature.
- Educate the parents regarding skin care (e.g. avoidance of harsh soaps, frequent bathing, using water rather than baby wipes).
- Check the eyes for any discharge – take a swab if appropriate and refer for treatment.
- Examine the mouth for any signs of infection (e.g. white spots may be sign of oral thrush).

- Check the shape of the head, and position of the eyes and ears. Patent nostrils or fontanelles for bulging or depression. Note any moulding, trauma or caput. Measured during initial examination.
- Examine the palate, ideally using a pen light and tongue depressor. A cleft palate or lip may lead to the baby being unable to feed, become dehydrated and fail to develop. During feeding, the baby may not latch correctly, a clicking sound may be heard or nasal regurgitation may occur.
- Check for any tongue ties and refer if found or suspected.
- Check that the limbs and digits are present and moving normally. Check for webbing between digits and for presence of nails, any paronychia.
- Check foot alignment for any talipes. Refer to a paediatrician if suspected.
- Examine the baby for any sins of IUGR.
- Examine the cord/umbilical area. Is the cord on or off, dry, not sticky? There should be no odour or inflammation. If needed, take a swab. Advise the mother to keep the nappy off the cord, especially in boys, to minimise contamination from urine and faeces. Remove the cord clamp as per Trust policy.
- Examine the nappy area for any soreness or discharge.
- Discuss with the mother about the frequency of wet and soiled nappies and colour of the stool passed.
- Weigh the baby if appropriate – newborn babies will commonly lose up to 10% of their birth weight during the first 7 days. Any greater weight loss or continued weight loss must be followed up.

- Undertake any neonatal screening as required – in some Trusts a baby's pulse oximetry is conducted while in hospital.
- Support the parents with any baby care queries (e.g. changing nappies, cord care, bathing baby).
- Document findings.

Source: Ewer, A.K., Middleton, L.J., Furmston, A.F. et al. (2011) Pulse oximetry screening for congenital heart defects in newborn infants (PulseOx): a test accuracy study. Published online 5 August at www.thelancet.com.

Newborn and infant physical examination (NIPE)

NB: The additional elements performed during this full examination *must* only be undertaken by a fully trained and qualified NIPE practitioner – either a midwife or a paediatrician. Much of the examination overlaps with the routine checks performed at birth and over the subsequent postnatal visits, but this screening is more detailed. It is not possible to provide full details within this book; therefore practitioners should always refer to additional sources of information where needed.

The examination is undertaken within the first 72 hours and again at 6–8 weeks with key elements of examination of eyes, heart, neurological, hips and testes/genitalia. Full guidance can be found in the newborn and infant physical examination (NIPE) screening programme (Public Health England 2019).

Key principles

- Inform the parents about what to expect and any findings.
- Refer any deviations from the normal and provide a follow-up plan.
- Obtain consent.
- Document detailed findings.
- Where a baby is premature, conduct the tests when the baby's condition permits.
- Gather a complete history (e.g. obstetric history, type of birth, medications, etc.).

Screen positive

The following timeframes are recommended where a baby screens positive for any conditions:

- Eye screen positive – opthalmology review in 2 weeks.
- Heart screen positive – senior paediatrician review before home. Urgency depends on condition.
- Hip screen positive – hip ultrasound by 2 weeks of age.
- Hip risk factors present – ultrasound by 6 weeks.
- Bilateral undescended testes – consultant paediatrician/ associate assessments within 24 hours of NIPE.
- Unilateral undescended testis – GP review at 6–8 weeks.

EYE

Approximately 2–3 in 10,000 babies have congenital cataracts. Risk factors include family history, genetic syndromes, extensive port wine staining, maternal viral exposure in pregnancy, neuro-developmental conditions or sensorineural hearing loss, prematurity. Causes of eye problems can include, for example, excessive vitamin A intake, exposure to rubella, CMV, syphilis, cocaine, alcohol consumption in pregnancy.

Procedure

- The mother's recent obstetric history and the family history of a first-degree relative with an ocular condition which was congenital or developed in early childhood (particularly congenital cataracts).
- Wash hands and gain consent.

- Assess the appearance of the eyes (external examination) for the ability to fully open the eyelids, both eyes and pupils the same size and symmetrical, pupils are round.
- Assess clarity of the cornea (the cornea diameter in a term baby should be similar to the width of the practitioner's little fingertip). Refer if signs of congenital cataracts, as this requires prompt surgery.
- Check for congenital glaucoma. This affects around 1 in 10,000 babies and occurs due to a failure to drain fluid away caused by damage within the eye. Can be inherited. The baby is often sensitive to light with cloudy, watery eyes.
- Check for signs of jaundice – yellow sclera or white flecks in the iris – trisomy 21.
- Examine for the red reflex with the overhead lights switched off or dimmed and the baby settled.
- Hold the eyepiece of the ophthalmoscope up to the baby's eye, at arm's length from their face. Direct the circle of light from the ophthalmoscope towards the baby's eye while gently parting the baby's eyelids if necessary. The red reflex is viewed through the ophthalmoscope eyepiece. The colour, brightness and presence of any shadows on the red reflex should be noted in each eye. A white reflex is abnormal.

Result: Caucasian babies have a bright, pinky-red reflex. The reflex can be less bright and of yellow/brown/orange hue in non-Caucasian babies. It may be helpful to assess the parents' red reflexes to determine the expected reflex colour.

- Refer any abnormalities for opthalmology follow-up appointments and document findings.

- Educate the parents to observe for problems such as nystagmus, asymmetry of the eye.
- If screening is clear transfer to the healthy child programme.

HEART

The overall incidence of congenital heart disease (CHD) is about 8 in 1000 babies (range 6 to 12 per 1000 live births). Critical congenital heart disease (CCHD) accounts for 15 to 25% of these and is a leading cause of morbidity and mortality. Babies reported as becoming cyanosed during feeds may have some form of heart problem.

Risk factors include the following:

- Family history of CHD in first-degree relative.
- Fetal trisomy 21 or other trisomy diagnosed.
- Cardiac abnormality suspected from the antenatal scan.
- Maternal exposure to viruses, such as rubella during early pregnancy.
- Maternal conditions, such as diabetes (type 1), epilepsy, systemic lupus erythematosis (SLE).
- Drug-related teratogens during pregnancy, including antiepileptic and psychotrophic drugs.

Procedure

- Obtain the mother's medical and recent obstetric history, including any medication.
- Obtain the baby's family history and ascertain current well-being.

- Ask the parents if the baby ever gets breathless or changes colour at rest or when feeding, has normal feeding behaviours and energy levels (e.g. is over too tired to feed, quiet, lethargic), or has poor muscle tone.
- Check the baby for general tone, central and peripheral colour, size and shape of chest, respiratory rate.
- Observe symmetry of chest movement, use of diaphragm and abdominal muscles and for signs of respiratory distress (recession/grunting).
- Undertake palpation of the femoral and brachial pulses for strength rhythm and volume.
- Assess perfusion through capillary fill time.
- Palpate the position of the cardiac apex (to exclude dextrocardia).
- Palpate the liver to exclude hepatomegaly (may be present in congestive heart failure).
- Examine for any vibratory sensation felt on the skin (+/– thrill).

Auscultation

NB: Use both the bell and diaphragm sides of the stethoscope at each point.

- Second intercostal spaces adjacent to the sternum: left (pulmonary area).
- Second intercostal spaces adjacent to the sternum: right (aortic area).
- Lower left sternal border in the fourth intercostal space (tricuspid area).
- Apex (mitral area).
- Midscapulae (coarctation area).

Following assessment

- If no abnormalities found transfer to the healthy child programme.
- Educate the parents to contact medical help if the baby shows any abnormal signs.
- If a problem is identified refer to a *senior* paediatrician. Urgency of referral will depend on the condition suspected.

Abnormal signs

Tachypnoea when resting, apnoea more than 20 seconds with colour change (e.g. cyanosis, sternal recession, nasal flaring, central cyanosis, absent or weak femoral pulses, presence of murmurs/extra heart sounds).

NB: Murmurs are classed as significant if they are loud, cover a wide area, exist in the presence of other abnormal findings or sound harsh in nature. Many babies will have a murmur for the first 24 hours. Other babies with cardiac anomalies may present with no murmur.

Some babies will present with a short, soft, systolic murmur around the left sternal border which is typically benign. Should any murmur be identified it should be discussed with a senior paediatrician ideally with cardiac expertise.

NEUROLOGICAL EXAMINATION

Prior to undertaking this part of the examination make sure you revisit the anatomy and physiology of the nervous system to help your understanding.

Always make sure parental consent is obtained and a full history is obtained. Consider the whole picture.

Refer any deviations from the normal.

This element of the neonatal assessment checks for 8 reflexes as follows:

Sucking reflex – Develops from the cranial nerves V, VII, IX, X and XII and from 28 weeks' gestation. A newborn should automatically suck at anything touching the roof of its mouth.

Rooting reflex – When stroking a baby's cheek it should turn its head and open its mouth.

Palmar grasp – If palm is stimulated the baby will grasp a finger. Grasp is harder when the finger is withdrawn.

Babinski reflex – When the sole of the foot is firmly stroked the big toe raises up and the other toes spread.

Tonic neck reflex – When the baby is supine, and the head is turned to one side, the arm on the side the baby is facing will extend The opposite arm will flex.

Galant reflex (truncal incurvation reflex) – With the baby resting on the examiners hand, back uppermost, pressure applied down the spine causes the opposite side of the pelvis to flex towards the stimulus.

Moro reflex (startle reflex) – The baby is supported under the head and shoulders off the surface with the arms held flexed across the baby's chest. When released to drop back the baby will respond to the lack of support by extending and abducting its arms, then returning them. The hands will open and the fingers form a C shape. The baby will often cry.

EXAMINATION OF THE HIPS

Approximately 1 or 2 in 1000 babies have hip problems that require treatment. Early detection and referral can minimise the risk of the need for surgery or long-term complications such as reduced mobility. 1–3% of babies can be found with developmental dysplasia of the hip, and 80% of girls and 20% of babies will have bilateral displacement.

Undetected unstable hips with delayed treatment may result in the need for complex surgery and/or long-term complications such as reduced mobility and pain and osteoarthritis.

Risk factors

- First-degree family history of hip problems in early life.
- Breech presentation at or after 36 completed weeks of pregnancy, irrespective of presentation at birth or mode of delivery even with a successful ECV. Or breech presentation at the time of birth between 28 weeks' gestation and term.
- Multiple pregnancy.
- Referral for an ultrasound scan should be arranged if any of these risk factors are present as deemed appropriate. Consultation with an experienced clinician is recommended.
- Isolated clicky hips do not require an USS and should be recorded as 'other' on S4N.

Procedure

- Obtain full history, obstetric, family and for risk factors.
- Obtain consent.

- Ensure that hygiene and safety is maintained – a warm environment and on a firm, flat surface with the baby undressed and settled. Nappy removed.
- Observe posture and check that both legs can be separated equally without resistance.
- Hold legs extended to check for equal leg length and symmetry.

NB: Observation of skin creases for symmetry is no longer part of the NIPE screen 2019.

- Undertake Allis' sign (as shown in Figure 5). Are knees equal height when knees are flexed and feet are flat on the surface?

Figure 5 Demonstration of Allis' sign

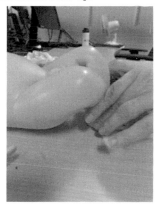

Ortolani's procedure to check for posterior dislocated hip. Each hip should be checked separately. The baby is supine and hip is flexed to 90 degrees and in a neutral position. While stabilising the opposite hip by cupping the hand around and placing the thumb on the symphysis pubis and fingers on the sacrum, the hip is *gently* abducted while lifting and pushing the femoral trochanter anteriorly. A palpable clunk is heard and felt when the hip proves positive for posterior dislocation.

- **CAREFUL** hand positioning is vital for this and Barlow's procedures. The thumb should be placed on the baby's inner thigh, opposite the lesser trochanter with the middle finger on the outer greater trochanter – avoid pressure on the knee (as shown in Figures 6, 7 and 8).

Barlow's procedure – This tests for dislocatable hips. Hips should be checked separately. Position hands and baby as for Ortolani's procedure (above). Without abduction push the leg back towards the table. If the hip can be dislocated a clunk will be felt as the head of the femur moves back out of the acetabulum.

If dislocation occurs – use Ortolani's procedure to reduce the dislocation.

- Refer if any positive Ortolani's or Barlow's for expert opinion within 4 weeks and USS within 2 weeks. If screening positive for risk factors and abnormal leg length but negative Ortolani and Barlow, refer for USS in 6 weeks and review by 8 weeks.
- Document findings in notes, red book and on NIPE Smart system.

Figure 6 Correct hand positioning for Ortolani's and Barlow's procedures

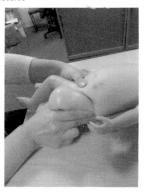

Figures 7 and 8 Abduction of the hip for Ortolani's procedure

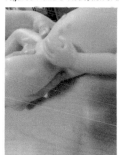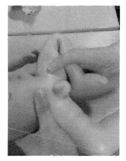

Figure 9 Position of leg for Barlow's procedure

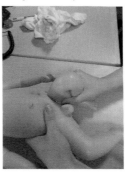

- Educate the parents to look out for and report if a click is heard, one leg appears longer than the other or is dragged when crawling, child walks with a limp or waddles, or legs cannot be abducted equally when changing nappies.

TESTES

Cryptorchidism (failure of the testes to descend) affects approximately 2–6% of male babies born at term and can lead to an increased risk of testicular cancer, reduced fertility, torsion and hypospadias. Bilateral undescended testes can be linked with ambiguous genitalia or endocrine disorder.

Risk factors include family history, low birth weight or SGA and prematurity.

Procedure

- Obtain consent and wash hands.

- Review history.
- Look for symmetry, size and colour.
- Palpate the scrotal sac to feel for the testes. If not located in the sacral sac feel for the testes in the inguinal canal. If found here and bilateral manage as a screen positive and record findings. Refer to be seen within 24 hours. If all normal, refer to the healthy child programme. If unilateral, review in 6–8 weeks.
- If identified at the 6- to 8-week, check to be seen by a senior paediatrician within 2 weeks.
- Check for any hydroceles. Common in newborns and often resolve spontaneously.
- Check for any hernias. Abnormal shapes or colour could indicate torsion of an inguinal hernia which requires prompt referral.
- Check the penis for any abnormal curvature (chordee), epispadias (urethral meatus develops on dorsal aspect), hypospadias (occurs on the ventral surface), webbing, buried or shortness in length.
- Check that the baby is passing urine.
- Document findings and refer as appropriate.

Girls

Though not part of the NIPE, female genitalia should be examined for any FGM (document clearly that this is absent at the time of examination), skin tags, secretions, bleeding, hymenal tags, ambiguity of the genitalia, groin swelling or fused labia.

It is vital to check that the baby is passing urine and that a full history is taken.

Neonatal jaundice

Jaundice is the most common condition that may require medical attention in newborns: 60% term and 80% pre-term babies will develop jaundice. Jaundice is the result of the accumulation of unconjugated bilirubin which leads to yellow coloration of the skin and mucous membranes. In most infants this is not a problem, but in some infants serum bilirubin levels may rise excessively, which can be harmful. Unconjugated bilirubin is neurotoxic and can, if excessive and not treated, cause death in newborns and lifelong neurologic problems in infants who survive. These babies may develop kernicterus.

Physiology (a brief description)

Neonatal jaundice develops as a result of the breakdown of the excess fetal red blood cells, no longer required after birth, into haem and globin. There is also a simultaneous change of cell haemoglobin from fetal to adult haemoglobin. The haem component is reduced into unconjugated bilirubin, which is fat soluble and requires proteins to transport it to the liver for disposal. If this protein is absent there is a risk that unconjugated bilirubin can remain in the circulation and cross into the brain.

If proteins are present, the unconjugated bilirubin is transported to the liver and converted by enzymes into water-soluble bilirubin. This is transported to the small intestine via the bile ducts, followed by the colon. The waste products from this process are excreted in the urine and faeces, giving them their colour.

■ PHYSIOLOGICAL JAUNDICE

At birth the liver is immature and intestinal function is decreased until feeding is established. Subsequently breastfed babies may be more prone to longer periods of jaundice (breastfeeding jaundice).

The degree of jaundice can also be affected by gestational age and also by the degree of trauma suffered at birth. Bruising from an instrumental birth, for example, can further increase the amount of bilirubin produced.

Signs and symptoms

- Develops from around day 3.
- Slowly disappears after 5 days.
- The baby is usually well and feeding regularly.
- Generally begins on the face and spreads downwards.
- Yellow coloration of the sclera of the eyes and mucous membranes (e.g. gums).

Assessment and management

- Explore history of birth, pregnancy, etc. for any predisposing factors.
- Examination should be conducted in good natural light.
- Assess overall well-being – tone, alertness, bowel and bladder function. Check blanched skin.
- Examine the face, body skin, gums and tongue for yellowing (consider ethnicity).
- Obtain a capillary serum bilirubin sample if considered appropriate. If high, then treatment may be required – see section on phototherapy (p. 57).

- Management depends on severity – monitor and review regularly/screen/transfer/treat.
- Educate the parents about signs and symptoms.
- If the baby is otherwise well – regulate feeds to 3–4 hourly, waking the baby if required.
- Supplementary feeds or extra fluids are *not* recommended for breastfed babies.

■ PATHOLOGICAL JAUNDICE

- Possible causes include haemolytic disease, rhesus disease, ABO incompatibility, genetic links (e.g. trisomies 13,18 and 21), metabolic disorders, infection (e.g. toxoplasmosis).
- Increased risk for premature babies or those with underlying conditions.
- Develops within the first 2 days of life.
- High levels of unconjugated bilirubin develop and can lead to kernicterus.
- Needs immediate referral and treatment.

Signs of Kernicterus/bilirubin encephalopathy

Greatest blood supply to areas damaged first – blood brain barrier is disrupted so damage to basal ganglia, brainstem, auditory, ocular nuclei. Serum bilirubin >340 micromol/litre in term baby is damaging or a rapid rise of >8.5 micromol/litre per hour.

- Hypotonia followed by poor sucking reflex, poor feeding.
- Lethargy, unresponsiveness.
- Fitting.
- Irritability/high pitched cry.

- Back arching.
- Vomiting.

Treatment

- Phototherapy.
- Intravenous immunoglobulin (IVIG) with multiple phototherapy.
- Double-volume exchange transfusion.
- Administer any medication (e.g. antibiotics).
- Regular serum bilirubin checks.
- Provide reassurance to parents.
- Regular observations, hygiene and feeding as per protocol/medical advice.
- Documentation.

■ PHOTOTHERAPY

Bilirubin is altered by exposure to light. Therefore, exposing a jaundiced baby to light will aid the breakdown of harmful unconjugated bilirubin.

Phototherapy will be commenced when blood serum levels of bilirubin are high. This is determined using graphs.

Access NICE (2010, updated 2016) treatment threshold graphs Guideline 98, and Trust guidance, which provide ranges for different gestations. (Further information may be found in the Neonatal Jaundice guideline by the National Collaborating Centre for Women's and Children's Health.)

- Equipment can either produce blue or white wave light with different effects.

- Overhead units or specially designed cots can be used. Extreme jaundice may require double phototherapy or even a blood exchange transfusion.
- Side effects can include raised temperature, watery stools, retinal damage, rashes and dehydration.

Care of a baby undergoing phototherapy

- The light source *must* be a safe distance from the baby (screens/head shields will be used).
- The baby's eyes should remain covered with goggles whenever the light source is on.
- Regular monitoring of the baby's temperature.
- The baby is likely to be nursed naked except for a nappy.
- Regular checks of serum bilirubin. Turn lights off to take sample.
- Maintain hygiene, especially around nappy and cord areas in light of frequency of passing loose stools.
- Prevent infection.
- Encourage bonding with parents whenever possible – provide reassurance.

Neonatal screening

■ HEARING TESTS

Hearing problems are estimated to affect 1–3 in 1000 babies. It is recommended that all newborn babies are now given a hearing test prior to discharge from hospital or have the test as soon as possible when home. The two non-invasive tests (the oto-acoustic emission and automated auditory brainstem response test) measure emissions of low-level inaudible sounds from the inner ear. The benefit of such early screening lies in the early intervention of speech therapy in those found to have hearing impairment.

■ SERUM BILIRUBIN

A capillary blood sample from the baby's heel, which tests for the level of serum bilirubin. The result is plotted on a graph and a decision made whether to use phototherapy or not. (See the jaundice and phototherapy sections, pp. 54 and 55.) Once taken, the sample should be labelled and covered before being forwarded to the laboratory. This minimises the exposure to light which causes the breakdown of the bilirubin content, leading to an inaccurate result.

■ NEONATAL BLOOD SPOT

- Undertaken between 5 and 8 days when feeding is more established (day of birth is commonly counted as day 0). Make sure that the baby feels secure by cuddling or feeding during the procedure.
- Screens for all or some of the following – phenylketonuria (PKU), congenital hypothyroidism (CHT), cystic fibrosis

(CF), altered haemoglobins (e.g. sickle cell) and MCADD (medium-chain acyl-CoA dehydrogenase deficiency), phenylketonuria, maple syrup urine disease, isovaleric acideamia, glutaric aciduria type 1 and homocystinuria.

- Post to laboratory within 24 hours of sample being taken.
- For more information refer to Standards and Guidelines for Newborn Blood Spot Screening (2019). UK Newborn Screening Programme Centre. www.newbornbloodspot.screening.nhs.uk.

NB: The Blood Spot Card is periodically updated; go to the following link for the current version in use: www.newbornbloodspot.screening.nhs.uk/bloodspotcard.

NB: When taking the sample ensure that the card does not come into contact with the foot or is dabbed several times to fill the circles.

Procedure

- Obtain and document consent from the parents.
- Complete all boxes on the card and apply the baby's barcode label (when available). If the label is unavailable the NHS number *must* be written on the card.
- Avoid contamination when completing the card.
- Ensure that the baby is held either by a parent or the midwife, in a secure position. Having the legs hanging downwards can help blood flow. Breastfeeding during the procedure can alleviate some distress.
- Clean and warm the heel. Use a warm towel or pad. *Do not* immerse in hot water to avoid risk of scalding.
- Wash hands and put on gloves.

Figure 10a Sample of a Blood Spot Card (front)

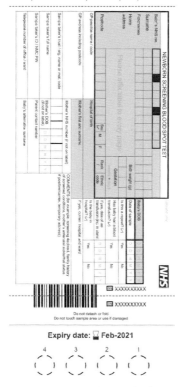

Expiry date: Feb-2021

Figure 10b Sample of a Blood Spot Card (back)

Baby's ethnic category		
	Code	Description
WHITE	A	British
	B	Irish
	C	Any other White background
MIXED	D	White and Black Caribbean
	E	White and Black African
	F	White and Asian
	G	Any other Mixed background
ASIAN	H	Indian
	J	Pakistani
	K	Bangladeshi
	L	Any other Asian background
BLACK	M	Caribbean
	N	African
	P	Any other Black background
OTHER	R	Chinese
	S	Any other ethnic category
	Z	Not stated

RANK
Identifies birth order: singleton, twins, triplets
1/1 Singleton   1/2 Twin 1   2/2 Twin 2   1/3 Triplet 1   etc

BLOOD COLLECTION
ALL fields on the card must be completed. Full blood spot
sampling guidelines for newborn screening are available from
www.gov.uk/government/publications/newborn-blood-spot-screening-
sampling-guidelines

☑ CORRECT	☒ INCORRECT	
Circle filled and soaked through to the back of the card	Layering	Insufficient multiple application
	Compressed	Insufficient small volume spots

IVD ② ⚠ CE 🛈   PerkinElmer Health Sciences, Inc.
72 P and N Drive, Greenville, SC 29611 USA

Expiry date: ⌛ Feb-2021   EC REP   Emergo Europe, Prinsessegracht 20,
2514 AP The Hague, The Netherlands

PerkinElmer 226 Ahlstrom LOT 110092 / 3024000x

○ ○ ○ ○ ○ ○ ○ ○ ○

1   2   3   4

Source: UK Newborn Screening Programme Centre www.newbornbloodspot.
screening, nhs.uk/bloodspotcard. Reproduced with permission.

Figure 11 Correct sites for obtaining blood samples from the baby's heel

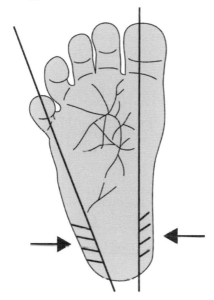

- Using an automated lancet, prick the heel once. A repeat stab (in a different place) should only be performed if bleeding is insufficient.

- Heel puncture should be performed on the plantar surface of the heel (as shown in Figure 11) to minimise trauma.
- Wait up to 15 seconds to allow blood to flow.
- Apply the blood drop to one side of the card. Do not touch the foot onto the card.
- Allow the blood to fill the circle by natural flow, and seep through to the back. Fill the circle completely and avoid layering.
- Wipe excess blood from the heel and apply gentle pressure to the wound with cotton wool to stem bleeding. Apply a spot plaster and advise the parents to remove it no later than 24 hours afterwards or immediately if any signs of an allergic reaction occurs.
- Dispose of sharps and clinical waste.
- Remove gloves and wash hands.
- Sign the form and insert into the envelope provided. Post the card within 24 hours.
- Document the test number and date in the postnatal records.
- Inform the parents how they will hear about the results. Results are usually sent through to GP clinics or health visitors who will transfer the results to the 'red book'. If any abnormalities are detected the parents will be contacted via the hospital and the baby brought back for repeat tests.

TIP

If bleeding stops during the procedure firmly wipe across the puncture site with gauze or cotton wool. Only if needed, repeat the puncture with a clean lancet on a different part of the foot.

Post birth care

■ INITIAL GENERAL CARE (IN NO PARTICULAR ORDER)

- Provide adequate analgesia.
- Stop any infusions when permitted to do so.
- Remove any cannulas and epidural tubing when safe to do so.
- Assist with hygiene – help into the shower/bedbath.
- Assist with initial feed – encourage skin-to-skin even if not intending to breastfeed.
- Ensure that urine is passed within 4 hours post birth.
- Assess vital signs – BP, pulse, temperature. Frequency will depend on maternal well-being and mode of delivery.
- Palpate the uterus to ensure it is contracted.
- Provide refreshments.
- Check blood loss per vagina.
- Repair any perineal trauma and monitor regularly during the postnatal period.
- Check if bloods are required for Kliehauer if rhesus negative. Administer Anti D if required within the first 72 hours post birth.
- Educate the woman about reporting any problems.
- Answer any questions.
- Document findings.
- Act upon any deviations from normal.

■ POST INSTRUMENTAL

As above plus:

- Stronger analgesia may be required due to the greater likelihood of perineal trauma and discomfort.

- Physiotherapy referral may be appropriate to discuss postnatal exercises.

■ POST CAESAREAN SECTION

As above plus:

- Ensure that airway remains patent especially if post general anaesthetic.
- Continue oxygen therapy as prescribed.
- Refer to a physiotherapist to discuss breathing and abdominal exercises.
- Monitor the wound site for any oozing/bleeding. Apply a pressure dressing if needed.
- If a drain is *in situ* ensure that it is working correctly.
- Maintain a MEOWS chart and fluid balance chart.
- Provide adequate analgesia.
- Encourage mobility as soon as possible.
- It is likely that an intravenous infusion and catheter are *in situ* which will need monitoring and care.
- Gradually introduce fluids, then diet according to maternal condition.
- Apply elastic support stockings if not already *in situ*.
- Administer any prescribed heparin and/or antibiotics.
- Assist with caring for the baby as less mobile.

Subsequent postnatal examinations

After the initial care post birth regular examinations are undertaken.

- Read notes and birth summary.
- Wash hands and put on apron.

- Consider mental well-being – talk about how the woman is feeling/coping. Refer if any signs of a deterioration in mental health. Look for signs of baby blues/depression/psychosis.
- Observe the woman for general well-being – does she look pale, tired, unwell?
- Take vital signs – BP, pulse, respirations and temperature (the frequency of future recordings will depend on maternal condition and Trust policy). Not routine in the community unless indicated.
- Discuss method of feeding – ask how the breasts feel (e.g. are they engorged, tender, or has she got cracked nipples?) Observe a feed.
- Gently palpate the uterus to check that it is contracted and involution is taking place, if complaining of tenderness or heavier blood loss. No longer recommended on a routine basis (NICE 2015).
- Discuss the amount of vaginal loss. Ask to see the pads if concerned (see Lochia section, p. 3).
- If any perineal trauma occurred, visualise the wound site. Look for signs of inflammation, stickiness, infection. Refer for antibiotics and swab as appropriate.
- If post Caesarean section – examine wound for signs of healing. (Remove sutures/clips if and when appropriate.)
- Discuss bladder function. If policy, collect and measure the first urine output following the birth.
- Discuss bowel function. Constipation can be common following a birth, especially if taking regular analgesia. Encourage intake of fluid and fibre in diet. May need a mild laxative.

- Examine legs for any signs of thrombosis or excessive oedema. Advise re exercise and elevation of legs when sitting. Ensure that the mother rests. Refer if sign of DVT.
- Record all findings in postnatal notes/MEOWS charts.
- Act on any deviations from normal.

Table 3 Postnatal complications

COMPLICATION	COMMENTS
Breast engorgement	• Occurs as milk production takes over from colostrum production. More milk than can be stored in the acini cells is initially produced, which leaks into the surrounding breast tissue • Occurs in all women following childbirth, irrespective of feeding method, from around day 3 • Women may experience discomfort and develop a pyrexia • Mild analgesia such as Paracetamol × 1 gram can help with both of these symptoms. (No more than 8 tablets in 24 hours) • Women should wear a well-fitting and supportive bra • If ceasing breastfeeding, avoidance of breast stimulation is beneficial. Otherwise encouraging the baby to feed will help

Table 3 (Continued)

COMPLICATION	COMMENTS
	• If heavily engorged, women may find attaching the baby to the breast more difficult. Hand expressing a small amount of milk should soften the breast to aid attachment • The use of cabbage leaves and hot/cold flannels is not supported by scientific evidence; however, women sometimes find them of benefit
Sore/cracked nipples	• Usually due to incorrect attachment during feeds • Check the baby's attachment and reposition if needed • Creams may relieve some of the discomfort between feeds
Mastitis	• Usually occurs due to inadequate emptying of the breast, alongside pressure from an incorrectly attached baby or ill-fitting bra. Blockages in the milk ducts can become infected, leading to pain, redness and lumps forming • Feeding baby regularly and ensuring correct attachment will help • If the symptoms persist, then antibiotics may be required

(Continued)

Table 3 (Continued)

COMPLICATION	COMMENTS
Pain/perineal discomfort	• The degree of pain depends on the individual and the mode of birth/degree of any trauma • Mild analgesics (e.g. Paracetamol), if taken regularly, can help and most are safe if breastfeeding. Stronger analgesics and anti-inflammatories can be prescribed where appropriate • In some situations, cold packs can be useful. Bathing in warm water can also be soothing for perineal discomfort and will maintain hygiene • Avoidance of perfumed soaps, etc. and undertaking pelvic floor exercises will promote wound healing along with a healthy diet and adequate fluid intake • Uterine pain or painful stitches accompanied by inflammation or signs of infection must be followed up • To minimise the risks of sepsis women should be encouraged to wash their hands before and after changing pads and using the toilet
Deep vein thrombosis	• Childbearing women have a much higher risk of developing a DVT • Most commonly situated in the legs • Signs and symptoms include localised swelling, inflammation and pain

Table 3 (*Continued*)

COMPLICATION	COMMENTS
	• There is an increased risk of a clot travelling to the lungs, leading to pulmonary embolism – signs include breathlessness and chest pain • Refer to a medical practitioner as soon as symptoms develop • Prevention is best – encourage leg exercises, mobility, weight loss if needed and fluid intake. Avoid long journeys. Elastic support stockings can help
Urinary tract problems	• A degree of stress incontinence in the first few days following the birth is relatively common • Urinary tract infections should be ruled out if symptoms of frequency, burning or pain on micturition occur. (Note: urine will be mixed with lochia; therefore, if obtaining a mid stream urine sample, ask the woman to wash the vulval area thoroughly prior to collection) • Encourage fluid intake – aim for 2 litres of fluid per day • Woman should be encouraged to void urine within 4 hours of the birth or removal of a catheter. The amount of urine passed should be recorded

(*Continued*)

Table 3 (*Continued*)

COMPLICATION	COMMENTS
'Baby blues'	• Many women experience these from around the third to the tenth day post-partum • Usually self-limiting • Women can complain of tiredness, tearfulness and irritability • Extra reassurance and support from the midwife and family can help
Postnatal depression	• Can begin with signs of the 'baby blues' • Other symptoms include anxiety, lethargy, difficulty sleeping and feelings of guilt • Women with a history of depression, from low socioeconomic status or women who have experienced a traumatic labour and birth, are more at risk of postnatal depression • Requires referral as soon as possible
Puerperal psychosis	• Least common mental health condition, affecting around 1 in 500 women • Sudden onset after a period of feeling well • Women can demonstrate obsessional thoughts (e.g. their baby is dead) • Immediate referral is needed

Skin-to-skin

- Aim to initiate skin-to-skin within the first hour of birth to aid bonding and breastfeeding.
- Helps with maintaining the baby's temperature and regulation of the heartbeat.
- Can be undertaken by either parent.
- Especially beneficial for premature babies (kangaroo care).
- The baby should have direct skin-to-skin contact and then be covered with warm towels or blankets.

Sudden Infant Death Syndrome (SIDS)

■ ADVICE TO PARENTS

- Never smoke in the same room as the baby – preferably stop smoking. This includes both parents and family members.
- The baby should sleep on its back only. To avoid flattening the occiput and problems with hip development parents are encouraged to keep the head in the midline when in a car seat and encourage play periods with the baby on its stomach.
- The baby's feet should be against the bottom of the cot.
- When indoors do not cover the baby's head.
- Avoid the baby overheating – add or remove single layers of natural fibre clothes if feeling cold or hot. Test the temperature by feeling the back of the neck or the abdomen rather than the forehead.
- Aim to have the baby sleeping in its parents' room for the first 6 months.
- Avoid sleeping in bed or on a chair with the baby, especially if under the influence of drugs, prescribed medication which could cause drowsiness or alcohol.
- If baby seems unwell seek medical help straight away.
- Breastfeed.
- Mattresses in cots should be of the appropriate standard.
- Avoid using cot bumpers, duvets and pillows when the baby is actually using the cot.

Support groups

Citizen's Advice Bureau 0344 411 1444
www.citizensadvice.org.uk.

Contact a Family for parents with/expecting disabled
children 020 7608 9700 info@contact.org.uk.

FSA Financial Services Authority 0805 111 6768
www.fsa.gov.uk.

Homestart 0116 464 5490 www.home-start.org.uk.

La Leche League breastfeeding advice and support
0345 120 2918.

Mental health www.mentalhealth-uk.org.

Miscarriage Association 0192 420 0799.

National Domestic Violence helpline 0808 802 3333.

NCT National Childbirth Trust 0300 330 0700.

NHS Direct 111.

NHS Drinkline www.nhs.uk/live-well/alcohol-support.

NHS Pregnancy Smoking Helpline 0300 123 1044.

Pregnancy loss and also mental health www.tommys.org.

SANDS Stillbirth and Neonatal Deaths 0808 164 3332
helpline@sands.org.uk.

TAMBA Twins and Multiple Births Association 0125 2332 344
www.tmba.org.uk.

Women aid general enquiries 0117 944 4411
www.info.womensaid.org.uk.

Working Families (Rights and Benefits) 0300 012 0312
www.workingfamilies.org.uk.

Thermoregulation of the newborn

Babies are at greater risk of losing heat due to a high surface area to body ratio, an immature heat regulatory centre, inability to shiver and low store of body fat. A low temperature will also impact upon the baby's ability to control its blood sugar. Babies with hypoglycaemia are also often hypothermic.

Routes of heat loss

- **EVAPORATION** – through moisture loss from wet skin.
- **CONVECTION** – heat drawn off by cool air passing over the skin.
- **CONDUCTION** – via direct contact with a cold surface.
- **RADIATION** – heat being lost to colder surfaces in close vicinity.

Avoid heat loss

- Shut windows and doors, and turn off fans during the birth and when performing any examinations to prevent draughts.
- Thoroughly dry the baby at birth and quickly dry after bathing.
- Do not place a baby directly onto cold surfaces (e.g. weighing scales). Use warm towels.
- Best of all, use skin-to-skin with mum or dad.

■ TRANSIENT TACHYPNOEA OF THE NEWBORN (TTN)

Occurs when the fluid found in the lungs in utero takes longer than expected to clear.

Symptoms

- Flaring of the nostrils.
- 'Grunting'.
- Sternal recession.

Action

- Refer to paediatrician.
- Observe and monitor for cyanosis.
- Screen for infection (surface swabs) if requested.
- Keep warm/monitor temperature.
- A capillary blood sugar may be requested.

References

EWER, A. K., MIDDLETON, L. J., FURMSTON, A. F. et al. (2011) Pulse oximetry screening for congenital heart defects in newborn infants (PulseOx): a test accuracy study. Published online 5 August at www.thelancet.com.

JOINT FORMULARY COMMITTEE (2020) British National Formulary. Available at www.medicinescomplete.com.

KNIGHT et al. (2019) *Saving Lives, Improving Mothers' Care*. Oxford: MBRRACE.

NATIONAL COLLABORATING CENTRE for WOMEN'S and CHILDRENS'S HEALTH (2010) *Neonatal Jaundice*. Available at http://nice.org.uk.

NATIONAL INSTITUTE for CLINICAL CARE EXCELLENCE (last updated 2015) *Postnatal Care up to 8 Weeks after Birth GC37*. London: NICE.

NATIONAL INSTITUTE for CLINICAL CARE EXCELLENCE (2010, updated 2016) *Treatment Threshold Graphs Guideline 98*. Available at http://nice.org.uk/guidance/CG98.

NURSERY and MIDWIFERY COUNCIL (2017) *Practicing as a Midwife in the UK*. London: NMC.

PUBLIC HEALTH ENGLAND (updated August 2019) *Newborn and Infant Physical Examination (NIPE) Screening Programme Handbook*. Available at www.gov.uk.

WHO/UNICEF (2016) *Protecting, Promoting and Supporting Breastfeeding: The Special Role of Maternity Services. A Joint WHO/UNICEF Statement*. Geneva: WHO.

Student Notes
